M000026614

WHEN WAS THE LAST TIME?

QUESTIONS TO EXERCISE THE MIND

Matthew Welp

authorHOUSE®

AuthorHouse™
1663 Liberty Drive
Bloomington, IN 47403
www.authorhouse.com
Phone: 1 (800) 839-8640

© 2016 Matthew Welp. All rights reserved.

No part of this book may be reproduced, stored in a retrieval system, or transmitted by any means without the written permission of the author.

Published by AuthorHouse   04/06/2016

ISBN: 978-1-5049-8700-4 (sc)
ISBN: 978-1-5049-8698-4 (hc)
ISBN: 978-1-5049-8699-1 (e)

Library of Congress Control Number: 2016904769

Print information available on the last page.

Any people depicted in stock imagery provided by Thinkstock are models, and such images are being used for illustrative purposes only. Certain stock imagery © Thinkstock.

This book is printed on acid-free paper.

Because of the dynamic nature of the Internet, any web addresses or links contained in this book may have changed since publication and may no longer be valid. The views expressed in this work are solely those of the author and do not necessarily reflect the views of the publisher, and the publisher hereby disclaims any responsibility for them.

The most important thing with these questions
is to enjoy the journey for the answers.

When was the last time you made a paper airplane?

When did you last take your temperature?

When did you last climb a ladder?

When was the last time you put on insect repellent?

When did you last drink lemonade?

When was the last time you adjusted the volume on something?

When were you last on a farm?

What was the last email you sent?

When was the last time you yawned?

When did you last shoot a squirt gun?

When did you last go up stairs?

When did you last speak to a pharmacist?

When was the last time you jumped rope?

Where was the last place you had to wait in a line?

What did you see the last time you went to the circus?

When did you last eat cereal?

When was the last time you saw a pocket watch?

When did you last write something using your non-dominant hand?

When was the last time you saw lightning?

When were you last in a pet store?

What was the last movie you watched?

When was the last time you bought a belt?

When was the last time you rang a doorbell?

When was the last time you held your breath?

What was the last thing you threw in the trash?

When did you last squeeze a piece of fruit to see if it was ripe?

When did you get your last toothbrush?

When was the last time you slept in a tent?

When was the last time you walked up a ramp?

When did you last use plastic silverware?

When was the last time you saw fireworks?

When did you last drink tea?

What was the last black and white photograph you saw?

When did you last vote?

When was the last time you covered your ears because something was too loud?

How did you get your last bruise?

When was the last time you had to provide your Social Security number?

When did you last use an electric pencil sharpener?

What was the last thing you pointed at?

When was the last time you saw a parade?

When did you last ride the bumper cars?

When was the last time you spoke into a microphone?

When did you last eat at a Chinese restaurant?

What was the last thing you had to chase because the wind was carrying it away?

When did you last touch your ear with your hand?

When did you last use a stapler?

When was the last time you dipped a chip?

When did you last pack a suitcase?

When was the last time you listened to your favorite song?

When did you last see a school bus?

When was the last time you shaved?

When was the last time you blew out a candle?

When did you last use a calculator?

When was the last time you opened a bathroom drawer?

When was the last time you were in a building over 3 stories tall?

When was the last time you adjusted the thermostat?

When did you last exercise?

When was the last time you roasted a marshmallow?

What was the last word you spelled out loud?

When did you last see a rabbit?

What was the last concert you attended?

When was the last time you whispered?

When did you last peel an orange?

When was the last time you threw a coin into a fountain?

When was the last time you had something stuck in your eye?

When was the last time you felt dizzy?

When was the last time you danced?

When did you last build a snowman?

When was the last time you watched television?

Who was the last person you talked to about the weather?

How did you last burn your tongue?

When did you last get new shoes?

What was the last thing you got from a vending machine?

When was the last time you opened the refrigerator?

When did you last use Velcro?

When was the last time you had a drink with ice in it?

When was the last time you carved a pumpkin?

When did you last eat cake?

When did you last roll dice?

When was the last time you whistled?

When was the last time you felt something in your shoe?

When did you last hear someone snore?

Who was the last person you saw wearing a hat?

When did you last get someone's autograph?

When was the last time you played cards?

When did you last go to an art museum?

When was the last time you used an ice pack?

When was the last time you blew bubbles?

When was the last time you took a bath?

When did you last check for dust by swiping your finger across something?

When was the last time you ate pancakes?

When was the last time you wore a life jacket?

When was the last time you stretched?

What was the last present you gave?

When was the last time you used a lighter?

When was the last time you ate at an all-you-can-eat buffet?

When was the last time you used a take-a-penny, leave-a-penny tray?

When did you last hear wind chimes?

When was the last time you ate french fries?

When was the last time you gave money to a street performer?

When was the last time you were in a hospital?

When did you last have your vision checked?

When was the last time you ate soup?

What was the last picture you took?

When did you last hear popcorn popping?

When did you last see a cow?

When was the last time you used a plunger?

When was the last time you heard the word <u>thaw</u>?

What was the last article of clothing you bought?

When was the last time you used a rubber band?

When was the last time you went through an automatic car wash?

How did you celebrate last Thanksgiving?

When did you last play tic-tac-toe?

When was the last time you made a snow angel?

When did you last see a windmill?

When did you last wear sweatpants?

When was the last time you ate a really good steak?

When was the last time you were bleeding?

When did you last bounce a ball?

When was the last time you heard a balloon pop?

When did you last hear someone speak a foreign language?

When did you last see a rainbow?

What was the last infomercial you watched?

When was the last time you ate a cookie?

When were you last at a shopping mall?

Where was the last place you forgot your jacket?

What was the last piece of trash you picked up off the ground?

When did you last sit in a massage chair?

When was the last time you painted?

When did you last see a police car?

When was the last time you popped bubble wrap?

When did you last eat pizza?

What was the last email you deleted?

When did you last drink water?

When was the last time you saw a clown?

When did you last hear the word <u>mug</u>?

When did you last go to the bathroom?

When was the last time you used a paper clip?

When did you last get a shot?

When was the last time you played hide-and-seek?

When were you last in a jewelry store?

When was the last time you watched a home movie?

When was the last time you blew your nose?

When was the last time you used a shovel?

When did you last do pushups?

When was the last time you were in a furniture store?

When was the last time you got a haircut?

When was the last time you used a cloth napkin?

When did you last fill a printer with paper?

When was the last time you wore something green?

What happened last Saturday?

When did you last get a paper cut?

When was the last time you heard a fire alarm?

What was the last movie you saw at the movie theatre?

When were you last on a college campus?

When was the last time you listened to classical music?

When did you last look through a photo album?

When did you last open a ketchup packet?

When was the last time you looked at a price tag?

When did you last adjust the speed of a ceiling fan?

When was the last time you ate a strawberry?

When did you last chew gum?

When was the last time you swung on a swing?

When was the last time you flipped a coin?

When was the last time you went to the zoo?

What was the last thing you got from the bottom shelf at the grocery store?

When was the last time you had the hiccups?

When was the last time you walked across a bridge?

How did you get your last scar?

When was the last time you went bowling?

When was the last time you used a key?

When did you last watch something with subtitles?

When was the last time you played rock, paper, scissors?

When did you last see a white horse?

When was the last time you boiled water?

When was the last time you used tweezers?

What was the last thing you plugged into a power outlet?

When was the last time you heard the word <u>sculpture</u>?

When was the last time you solved a maze?

When did you last look at a calendar?

What was the last present you wrapped?

When was the last time you heard a dog bark?

What was the last email you sent?

When was the last time you crossed your fingers?

Who was the last person you talked to about a book?

When was the last time you wrote something in cursive?

When was the last time you ate candy?

When was the last time you put a hood up over your head?

What happened last Wednesday?

When did you last cross a street?

When was the last time you took your pet to the veterinarian?

When was the last time you sat in a booth at a restaurant?

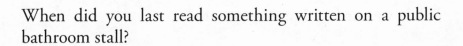

When did you last read something written on a public bathroom stall?

When was the last time you wore a hat?

When did you last close a window?

When did you last get a new coat?

Whose wedding did you last attend?

What was the last book you checked out from a library?

What was the last liquid you poured?

When was the last time you said out loud the number 9?

When did you last ride in a taxi?

When did you last write the date?

When was the last time you saw a cloud that reminded you of something?

When was the last time you pushed a shopping cart?

When was the last time you bought a rug?

When did you last check your mailbox?

What was the last idea you had for an invention?

How did you last get burned?

When was the last time you took leftovers home from a restaurant?

When did you last give a speech?

When was the last time you ate a donut?

When was the last time you heard the word <u>brag</u>?

When did you last jump on a trampoline?

When was the last time you stayed up all night?

When was the last time you stubbed your toe?

When did you last sit at a picnic table?

When was the last time you used a flashlight?

When was the last time you played bingo?

When was the last time you snapped your fingers?

Who was the last person you had a staring contest with?

When was the last time you went to the beach?

What room were you in before this one?

When did you last use pliers?

What was the last thing you bought?

When did you last have a different hairstyle?

How did you celebrate last Mother's Day?

When was the last time you cut your toenails?

When did you last eat at a Mexican restaurant?

When was the last time you skipped a stone on water?

What was the last text message you sent?

When was the last time you drank coffee?

When was the last time you cracked open an egg?

When did you last listen to the radio?

What was the last stain you got on your clothes?

When was the last time you noticed someone had a nose piercing?

Who was the last person to discuss religion with you?

When did you last work in a garden?

When was the last time you saw a lightning bug?

When did you last hear or see the price of gas?

When was the last time you winked?

What was the last spoken question you answered?

When did you last go down a slide?

When was the last time you flushed a toilet?

For what reason did you last use a saw?

What was the last item you returned for a refund?

What was the last billboard you read?

How did you last bump your head?

When was the last time you used a computer?

When did it last hail?

What was the occasion the last time you held a trophy?

When was the last time you saw someone smoking a cigarette?

What was the last knock-knock joke you heard?

When was the last time you were in a car for longer than one hour?

When was the last time you found out someone's middle name?

When did you last flip a light switch?

When was the last time you were in your high school?

When were you last in a bookstore?

Whose perfume or cologne did you last smell?

What was the last documentary you watched?

When was the last time you heard a car alarm?

What was the last thing you heated up in a microwave?

How did you celebrate last 4th of July?

When was the last time you checked the date?

What happened last Monday?

When did you last see a baseball field?

When did you last see a flag at half-staff?

When was the last time you saw an ambulance?

What was the last riddle you tried to solve?

When did you last put on a ring?

When was the last time you went for a walk?

When were you last in a candy store?

When was the last time you ate celery?

What was the last major decision you made?

When was the last time you had a headache?

When did you last go swimming?

When was the last time you were in a shoe store?

When was the last time you walked down stairs?

Who was the last person to tell you about a dream they had?

What was the last sporting event you watched on television?

What was the last balloon animal you saw someone make?

When was the last time you saw or heard what the temperature was outside?

When was the last time you clapped?

When was the last time you went through a haunted house?

When did you last eat an apple?

When was the last time you drew a picture of a house?

When did you last see a vehicle with its hazard lights on?

When was the last time you wore a button?

When was the last time you sneezed?

Where did you last ride in an elevator?

Who was the last person to shake your hand?

When was the last time you were farther than 1 mile from where you are right now?

What was the last voicemail you received?

When was the last time you looked at a clock?

When did you last shuffle playing cards?

When was the last time you donated clothes?

What was the last thing you got out of the freezer?

What was the last thing you typed into the Google search engine?

When was the last time you met someone who had the same first name as you?

When did you last drink hot chocolate?

When was the last time you put on perfume or cologne?

Who was the last person to tell you their name?

When was the last time you put on a necklace?

When was the last time you called a 1-800 number?

What was the last thing you heard about Germany?

When was the last time you played a lottery game?

When did it last rain?

When was the last time you drank wine?

What was the last thing you ate at an amusement park?

When was the last time you went through a revolving door?

When was the last time you used a salt shaker?

When was the last time you moved to a new home?

When was the last time you made a reservation at a restaurant?

What was the last thing you put in recycling?

When was the last time you got up during the night?

What was the last thing you bought that cost over $100?

When was the last time you went to a religious service?

When did you last see a motorcycle?

When did you last open a door?

When was the last time you used scissors?

When was the last time you washed the dishes?

When did you last feel like a word was on the tip of your tongue?

When was the last time you heard someone play the trumpet?

What was the last business card you took?

When was the last time you heard the word <u>dragon</u>?

When was the last time you used a measuring cup?

When was the last time part of your body was numb?

When did you last eat a hot dog?

When was the last time you put your hand in your pocket?

When were you last in a dollar store?

When was the last time you sat at a wobbly table?

When was the last time you went up an escalator?

When did you last lose a tooth?

When was the last time you spent the night away from home?

When was the last time you ate chocolate?

When was the last time you walked on grass?

When did you last see a $100 bill?

When was the last time you turned off a lamp?

When did you last work on a Sudoku puzzle?

When was the last time you finished a drink and there was ice left over?

When was the last time you went sledding?

When did you last see a bird?

When was the last time you looked through binoculars?

What was the last magazine you read?

When was the last time you threw a water balloon?

When was the last time you propped a door open?

When was the last time you got something out of someone else's refrigerator?

When was the last time you looked through a magnifying glass?

What was the last word you typed?

When was the last time you went to a casino?

When did you last use a kitchen sink sprayer?

Who was the last person you hugged?

When was the last time you pushed a wheelchair?

When was the last time you picked your nose?

What was the last cartoon you watched?

When was the last time you used a pencil?

When was the last time you touched a fire hydrant?

When was the last time you bought eggs?

When was the last time you washed your hands?

When was the last time you went ice skating?

Who was the last person you heard was pregnant?

When was the last time you saw a helicopter?

When was the last time you had to wait for a train to pass at a railroad crossing?

When was the last time you struggled to get a lid off?

When was the last time you were in a different state?

Who was the last person to hold your hand?

When was the last time you went through a drive-thru?

When was the last time you saw someone using sign language?

When was the last time you went into the toy section at a department store?

What was the last secret you were told?

When was the last time you opened a drawer in the kitchen?

When was the last time you used a crayon?

When was the last time you blew a whistle?

When was the last time you put on a Band-Aid?

What was the last thing you liked on Facebook?

When was the last time you were in a car accident?

What was the last board game you played?

When was the last time you answered someone else's phone?

When was the last time you walked on a hardwood floor?

When was the last time you ate turkey?

Who was the last person you talked to about their upcoming vacation?

When was the last time you broke a bone?

How did you celebrate last Christmas?

When was the last time you put syrup on something?

Who was the last person you added to your contacts on your cellphone?

When was the last time you ran into somebody you knew in an unexpected place?

When was the last time you adjusted the height of an office chair?

When was the last time you noticed you were wearing something that was reflecting light?

When was the last time you did the laundry?

When did you last buy a television?

What was the last mental calculation you did?

When was the last time you replaced the batteries in something?

When was the last time you played Scrabble?

When was the last time you got shocked?

When was the last time you were in a hot tub?

When was the last time you saw someone use crutches?

When was the last time you were in a car?

When was the last time you looked up the definition of a word?

When was the last time you weighed yourself?

When did you last buy a mattress?

When was the last time you cleaned the lenses on a pair of glasses?

When was the last time you drew a picture of a person?

When was the last time you went to Walmart?

When was the last time you picked up something that you saw someone else drop?

What was the last dream you had?

When was the last time you fell down?

When did you last wear boots?

Who was the last person to give you a tour of their house?

When was the last time your picture was taken by a professional photographer?

What was the last time you paid in cash?

When was the last time you cleaned the wax out of your ears?

When was the last time you checked your blood pressure?

When was the last time you heard the word <u>captain</u>?

When was the last time you had something scheduled at 10 am?

What was the last thing you said before you went to sleep last night?

When was the last time you bought a gift card?

When was the last time you muted a television?

When was the last time you slept on a couch?

When did you last speak to each of your family members?

When was the last time you had a blister?

When did you last get bit by a mosquito?

When was the last time you canceled an appointment?

What was the last thing you ate?

When was the last time you went roller skating?

When was the last time something got stuck in a tree?

When was the last time you couldn't find the remote?

When was the last time you saw the sunrise?

What did you last count?

When was the last time you pushed a stroller?

When was the last time you rode on a carousel?

What was the last musical you watched?

When was the last time you opened a window?

What was the last thing that got stuck in your teeth?

When was the last time you went to a family reunion?

What was the last word you wrote?

What happened on this day last year?

When was the last time you put on socks?

When was the last time you spoke to your neighbor on the right?

When was the last time you used a Ziploc bag?

When was the last time you took a nap?

When was the last time you felt someone's forehead to see if they had a fever?

When did you last use an ice scraper?

When was the last time you bought flowers?

When was the last time you wrote your signature?

When did you last brush your hair?

When was the last time you touched your nose with your hand?

When was the last time you heard someone say <u>needle in a haystack</u>?

When was the last time you used a phone that had a cord?

When was the last time you worked on a crossword puzzle?

When was the last time you walked a dog?

When was the last time your ears popped?

What was on the last grocery list you made?

When was the last time you heard bagpipes?

When was the last time you cleaned a mirror?

When did you last check the time?

When was the last time you tried exercise equipment at the store?

When was the last time you went trick-or-treating?

What was the last book you read?

When was the last time you moved something and found an outline of dust?

When did you last cough?

When was the last time you went up a mountain?

When was the last time you had a cavity?

What was the last drink you spilled?

When was the last time you heard the word <u>gallon</u>?

When was the last time you had something scheduled at 3 pm?

When was the last time you ate watermelon?

When was the last time you found money on the ground?

When was the last time you couldn't find your keys?

When did you last open a kitchen cupboard?

When was the last time you tried to think of a rhyme to a word?

When was the last time you ate carrots?

What was the last video game you played?

When was the last time you wished someone good luck?

When was the last time you flew a kite?

What was the last thing said to you?

When was the last time you read a newspaper?

When did you last have a nosebleed?

When was the last time someone tried to guess your age?

When was the last time you rode on a bus?

What was the last thing you stepped over?

When was the last time you got your picture taken behind a cutout?

When was the last time you were in a gym?

When was the last time you went fishing?

When was the last time you lit a match?

When was the last time you opened a garage door?

When did you last hear the word <u>yodel</u>?

When was the last time you wore gloves?

When did you last see an airplane in the sky?

When was the last time you used a Dustbuster?

When was the last time you were in a sporting goods store?

When was the last time you joined your hands behind your back?

When was the last time you jumped?

When was the last time you went to a graduation ceremony?

When did you last get a massage?

When was the last time you got brain freeze?

When was the last time you threw up?

When was the last time you heard a recording of your voice?

When was the last time you were in a casino?

What was the last thing you heard about Montana?

When was the last time you used a screwdriver?

Who was the last person you saw with a beard?

When was the last time you noticed a clock wasn't set right?

When was the last time you heard the word <u>treasure</u>?

When were you last outside?

What was the last thing you accidentally dropped?

When was the last time you donated money to charity?

When was the last time you ran the dishwasher?

When was the last time you gave someone a fist bump?

When was the last time you heard that someone had gotten engaged?

When did you last use a can opener?

When was the last time you ate ice cream?

When did you last sing?

What was the last article of clothing you tried on before you bought?

When was the last time you were on a dock?

When was the last time you put on shoes?

When was the last time you saw a bug?

When was the last time you went to the dentist?

How did you celebrate last Father's Day?

When was the last time you went through an automatic door?

When did you last put on a shirt?

When was the last time you saw a children's lemonade stand?

When did you last turn on a garbage disposal?

How did you celebrate your last birthday?

When did you last see a frog?

When was the last time you used a treadmill?

When did you last spend the night in a hotel?

When was the last time you opened a glove compartment?

When did you last address an envelope?

When was the last time you wore two outfits in one day?

When was the last time you sat around a fire pit?

What was the last thing you hung on the refrigerator?

When was the last time you hit a piñata?

When was the last time you gave someone a high five?

How did you celebrate last New Year's Eve?

When was the last time you watched the sunset?

When was the last time you went to a funeral?

What was the last thing you read on someone's shirt?

What was the last movie sequel you watched?

When was the last time you played Monopoly?

When was the last time you used chopsticks?

What was the last book you borrowed?

When was the last time you ate cheese?

What was the last thing you ate out of a bowl?

When was the last time you sang Happy Birthday to You?

When was the last time you raised your hand?

What was the last vacation you took?

When was the last time you heard the word gallop?

When was the last time you gave your credit card number over the phone?

When was the last time you used a broom?

When was the last time someone recorded a video of you?

What was on the last to-do list you made?

When was the last time you used glue?

What was the last movie preview you saw?

When was the last time you used a paddle?

When was the last time you looked through a brochure?

When was the last time you built a sand castle?

When was the last time you filled a pet's food dish?

When was the last time you saw someone wearing tie-dye?

When was the last time you met someone named Jenny?

When did you last put money in a parking meter?

What was the last thing you printed?

When was the last time you tied a knot?

When was the last time you went inside a gas station?

When was the last time you were tickled?

When did you last eat bacon?

When was the last time you were woken up by someone?

What was the last document you faxed?

When was the last time you stood up from a seated position?

When did you last hold a baby?

When were you last on a golf course?

When was the last time you used a garden hose?

When did you last hear glass break?

When was the last time you used Tupperware?

When was the last time you said the number 5 out loud?

When was the last time you looked at the stars?

When was the last time you bought sunglasses?

When was the last time you played checkers?

When did you last kick a soccer ball?

When was the last time you searched for Waldo?

What did your last fortune cookie say?

When was the last time you used a bathroom hand dryer?

When was the last time you used a GPS?

When was the last time you were late?

When did you last drink through a straw?

When was the last time you accidentally dialed a wrong number?

When did you last climb a tree?

When was the last time you used a coupon?

When was the last time it was over 100 degrees outside?

What was the last thing you ate with your hands?

When was the last time you blew up a balloon?

When did you last use a ruler?

When was the last time you heard the word <u>cactus</u>?

When was the last time you drank milk?

Where was the last place you parked your vehicle?

When was the last time you dropped someone off at the airport?

When was the last time you got a splinter?

When was the last time you felt hot?

What was the last music video you watched?

When was the last time you were on a boat?

When was the last time you ate a cupcake?

When did you last look at a menu?

When was the last time you pet a cat?

When did you last wave at someone?

When was the last time you saw a birdbath?

When was the last time you got a cramp?

When was the last time you lit a candle?

When did you last shovel snow?

When was the last time you stood in sand?

When did you last sleep in a sleeping bag?

When was the last time you used tape?

When was the last time someone took your picture?

When was the last time you took the garbage to the curb?

When was the last time you lost your voice?

When did you last pray?

When was the last time you did a word search?

When was the last time you played catch?

When did you last play solitaire?

When was the last time you held a stuffed animal?

When was the last time you ate food cooked on an outdoor grill?

When was the last time you touched something to see what it felt like?

When was the last time you ate a banana?

When was the last time you sat at your desk?

What was the last thing you said?

When was the last time you replaced a light bulb?

When was the last time you made a shadow puppet?

What was the last thing you bought online?

When was the last time you looked underneath your bed?

When was the last time you set an alarm clock?

What was the last bet you made?

What was the last thing you cooked in the oven?

When was the last time you went to Bed Bath & Beyond?

When was the last time you held a purse?

When was the last time you laughed so hard your abs hurt?

What was the last thing you memorized?

When was the last time you met someone named John?

When was the last time you couldn't find your cellphone?

Whose name did you last hear spoken aloud?

When was the last time you went to a water park?

When did you last open a window shade?

When was the last time you accidentally took a sip of someone else's drink?

When was the last time you ate broccoli?

When was the last time you played Candyland?

When was the last time you used a toaster?

When was the last time you flossed your teeth?

What was the last thing you wrote on a sticky note?

What was the last website you visited?

When was the last time you shopped for a greeting card?

When was the last time someone asked you how you wanted your eggs?

When was the last time you went to a museum?

When did you last recite the alphabet?

Who was the last person to touch your hair?

When was the last time you bounced a basketball?

When did you last put on a wristwatch?

When was the last time you looked through a telescope?

When was the last time you made the OK sign with your hand?

When was the last time you looked in a school yearbook?

When did you last hear someone give a toast?

What was the last DVD case you opened?

When was the last time you played Battleship?

What was the last thing you considered buying but didn't?

When was the last time you heard a song that you had never heard before?

When did you last drink from a Styrofoam cup?

When was the last time you used a zipper?

When was the last time you opened the cabinet door underneath the kitchen sink?

When was the last time you saw a lit fireplace?

When was the last time you ripped paper?

When was the last time you touched glass?

When was the last time something got stuck on the roof?

When was the last time your thumb and ring finger touched?

What was the last commercial you saw?

What was the last thing you heard about the governor?

When was the last time you looked through a lost-and-found box?

What was the last amusement park ride you rode?

When was the last time you did a connect-the-dots activity?

When was the last time you looked through the peephole of a door?

When was the last time you used a blender?

When was the last time you said out loud the number 4?

When did you last sit on a couch?

When was the last time you saw a wheelbarrow?

When was the last time you tied a shoe?

When was the last time you worked on a jigsaw puzzle?

When was the last time you pressed a button on a television?

When was the last time you sat on bleachers?

When was the last time you ate a sucker?

When was the last time someone you know got a new pet?

When was the last time you touched your feet with your hands?

When was the last time you turned on the fan in the bathroom?

When was the last time you had an allergic reaction?

When was the last time you wore jeans?

When was the last time you looked at the Nutritional Facts on food packaging?

When was the last time you had blood drawn?

When was the last time you rated something on a scale of 1 to 10?

When did you last see a turtle?

When did you last hold a beach ball?

When was the last time you put on deodorant?

When was the last time you cried?

When was the last time you read a book to a child?

When was the last time you noticed a faucet was leaking?

When did you last use your credit card?

When was the last time you ate fish?

When was the last time you went to the post office?

When was the last time you played tag?

When was the last time you went to a garage sale?

When was the last time you gave out your phone number?

Who was the last person to offer you a drink?

When did you last hear thunder?

What was the last password you created?

When was the last time you heard the word <u>bubble</u>?

When was the last time you heard a cricket?

When was the last time you wore someone else's shoes?

When did you last change the toilet paper roll?

When did you last use a clipboard?

When was the last time you used a travel-size tube of toothpaste?

When did you last change your diet?

When was the last time you cleaned out the inside of your vehicle?

When was the last time you tickled someone?

When did you last watch a cooking show?

When was the last time you played with a yo-yo?

When was the last time you ate an onion ring?

When was the last time you had a coughing fit?

When did you last buy socks?

When was the last time you used a locker?

When did you last touch a wall?

What was the last sticker you wore?

When was the last time you ate popcorn?

When was the last time you jammed your finger?

When did you last take a shower?

What was the last thing you bought that was on display in the checkout line?

When did you last take off your coat?

When was the last time you tried a free sample at the grocery store?

When was the last time the power went out?

When was the last time you were told to close your eyes?

When did you last hear a car horn?

When was the last time you put a leaf in a table?

When did you last hear someone talk in their sleep?

When did you last unwrap a present?

When was the last time you got a new Christmas ornament?

When did you last see a hot air balloon?

When was the last time someone asked you how to spell a word?

When did you last see a magic trick?

When did you last hear a gunshot?

When was the last time you read something on the back of a photograph?

When was the last time you ate outside?

When was the last time you stood on a chair?

When was the last time you noticed someone had braces?

When was the last time you slept on an inflatable mattress?

When did you last ride a bicycle?

When was the last time you heard a phone ring at a time when all phones should have been silenced?

When was the last time you wrote or typed your name?

When was the last time you traveled to another country?

When were you last in the newspaper?

When was the last time you dipped something in ketchup?

When was the last time you went in a photo booth?

Who was the last famous person you saw?

When was the last time you used a laptop?

When was the last time you lay in a hammock?

When did you last go out on a balcony?

When was the last time you heard about an earthquake, and where was it?

When was the last time you took a nap?

When was the last time you received a handwritten letter in the mail?

What was the last thing you put in the dirty laundry?

When was the last time you heard the phrase <u>last but not least</u>?

What was the last party you attended?

When was the last time you used an umbrella?

When did you last use jumper cables?

What was the last voice mail you left?

When did you last go to a carnival?

When was the last time you threaded a needle?

When did you last see someone do a cartwheel?

Who was the last person you saw wearing a suit?

When was the last time you closed a door?

How did you celebrate last Valentine's Day?

When was the last time you used a vacuum cleaner?

When did you last see a fire truck?

When was the last time you heard the word <u>scholarship</u>?

What was the last thing you smelled?

When did you last wear a scarf?

When was the last time you spit?

When was the last time you lay in the grass?

When was the last time you sat on a stool?

When was the last time you used a spoon?

When was the last time you crossed your legs?

When was the last time you got your hand stamped?

When was the last time you used a yellow highlighter?

When was the last time you hammered a nail?

Who was the last person you heard speak with an accent?

When was the last time you ate breakfast at a hotel?

When was the last time you mowed the lawn?

When were you last in a cellphone store?

When was the last time you used a fly swatter?

When was the last time you had a copy of a key made?

When was the last time you went down an escalator?

When were you last in a hardware store?

When was the last time you had the oil changed in your vehicle?

When was the last time you drank orange juice?

When was the last time you saw someone riding a skateboard?

When was the last time you wrote on a dry erase board?

When did you last put on sunscreen?

When was the last time you took an antibiotic?

When was the last time you wore a blue shirt?

When was the last time you used a VCR?

When was the last time you said your full name out loud?

When was the last time you heard The Star-Spangled Banner?

When was the last time you reclined in a chair?

When was the last time you opened the trunk of a vehicle?

When was the last time you watched a movie that was longer than 3 hours?

When was the last time you saw foreign currency?

When was the last time you used a public restroom?

When was the last time you drank from a drinking fountain?

What was the last email you received?

When was the last time you rolled up your sleeves?

When was the last time you plucked a hair?

When was the last time you wore a name tag?

When was the last time you ate at a table that had a tablecloth?

When did you last speak on the phone?

What was the last Halloween costume you wore?

When was the last time you hung something on the wall?

When was the last time you smelled cigarette smoke?

Who did you last see with hair dyed an unnatural color?

When did you last smell coffee?

When was the last time you turned on a lamp?

When was the last time you tore a paper towel from the roll?

In what order did you put on your clothes the last time you got dressed?

When was the last time you checked the size of an article of clothing?

When was the last time you wore headphones?

When was the last time you held a toothpick?

When was the last time you got something out of the linen closet?

What was the last class you took?

When was the last time you dialed 911?

When was the last time you went through a metal detector?

When was the last time you cleaned up broken glass?

When did you last use a colored pencil?

When was the last time you wore a cowboy hat?

When was the last time you locked a door?

When was the last time you used a rake?

Who is the newest member of your family?

When was the last time you helped someone move?

What was the last sound you heard?

When was the last time you were with a group of more than 10 people?

When were you last on a deck?

When was the last time you were in a bakery?

When was the last time you bought something at a meat counter?

When was the last time you smelled a scented candle?

When was the last time you reused a plastic grocery bag?

When did you last see smoke coming out of a chimney?

When was the last time you went through a tollbooth?

When was the last time you bought a picture frame?

When was the last time you paid for parking?

When was the last time you were part of a wedding party?

When did you last eat corn on the cob?

When was the last time you were in your childhood home?

When was the last time you played skee-ball?

When did you last see a soldier in uniform?

When did you last get new luggage?

When was the last time you held a feather?

When was the last time you went to a dance recital?

When was the last time you changed clothes in a car?

When was the last time you used a paper hole punch?

When did you last have food delivered?

When was the last time you drank a bottled water?

When was the last time you took your pulse?

When was the last time you spoke to an employee?

When was the last time you went shopping for a couch?

When was the last time someone you know was admitted to the hospital?

When did you last see the moon?

When was the last time you used a tape measure?

When was the last time you smelled a scratch and sniff?

What was the last thing you recorded on television?

What was the last thing you ate on an airplane?

When was the last time you noticed a house for sale?

When was the last time you saw a snake?

What was the last thing you threw?

When was the last time you played Connect 4?

When did you last eat pudding?

When was the last time you heard the word <u>volcano</u>?

When did you last test-drive a vehicle?

When was the last time you used hand sanitizer?

When did you last feel cold?

When was the last time you cut the tags off an article of clothing?

When was the last time you opened a can of pop?

When did you last hear a cat purr?

When was the last time you scratched an itch?

What was the last dessert you ordered?

When was the last time you rode on a ski lift?

When did you last play Go Fish?

When was the last time you sat on a porch?

When was the last time you held a door open for someone?

When did you last tuck in your shirt?

When was the last time you used a hair dryer?

When did you last wear a bathing suit?

What country's name did you last hear spoken aloud?

When was the last time you had diarrhea?

When did you last smell fresh bread?

When was the last time you stopped at a 4-way stop?

Who was the last person to talk to you about their pet?

When was the last time you complimented someone's hair?

When did you last hear the word <u>blush</u>?

When did you last see a butterfly?

When was the last time you used a pocketknife?

What was the last drawer you opened?

When was the last time you went to a park?

When was the last time you cleaned a stain out of carpet?

When was the last time you played chess?

When was the last time you scheduled to do something at 1 pm?

What happened last Thursday?

When was the last time you were in a gift shop?

When did you last donate blood?

When did you last turn on an electric fan?

What was the last personalized license plate you saw?

When was the last time you set the timer on the oven?

When did you last pull a weed?

When was the last time you told someone about a dream you had?

When was the last time you gave bunny ears to someone in a picture?

When was the last time you popped a pimple?

When was the last time you closed a bread bag?

What was the last thing you had engraved?

When was the last time you put on a belt?

When was the last time you wrote a dollar sign?

What was the last question you asked?

When was the last time you talked on the phone for more than 30 minutes?

When was the last time you crumpled a piece of paper into a ball?

When was the last time you cut a sandwich in half?

What was the last thing you wrote on a calendar?

When was the last time you ate a cheeseburger?

When was the last time you played miniature golf?

What was the last thing you got from a concession stand?

When was the last time you blew into your hand to see if your breath smelled bad?

When was the last time you hit rewind on a remote?

What was the last sporting event you attended?

When was the last time you were poked by a cactus?

When was the last time you accidentally threw away something important?

When did you last buy stamps?

When was the last time you got gum out of a gumball machine?

When was the last time you used the hidden key to get into your house?

What was the last thing you got out of your closet?

When was the last time you braided hair?

When did you last swing a baseball bat?

When was the last time you watered a plant?

When was the last time you cooked using a recipe?

When did you last have to find your seat by row letter and seat number?

When was the last time you used a crescent wrench?

When did you last yell for someone in another room?

When was the last time you gave someone a thumbs-up?

When was the last time you visited a nursing home?

When was the last time you went to a farmer's market?

When was the last time you sat on a porch swing?

When was the last time you brushed your teeth?

When was the last time the wind was so strong you could hear it?

When did you last open a folder?

When was the last time you were on a speedboat?

What was the last game show you watched?

When was the last time you saw a water tower?

When was the last time you rolled down a car window?

When was the last time you applied a cream to your skin?

What was the last jar you opened?

When was the last time you held a popsicle stick?

When was the last time you heard what someone's SAT or ACT score was?

Whose high school graduation party did you last attend?

When was the last time you drank root beer?

When was the last time you saw a police officer in uniform?

When was the last time you filled out a form that asked for your birthdate?

When was the last time you washed your face at a sink?

When was the last time you had to scribble with a pen to make it start writing?

When did you last see a stage curtain go up?

When were you last in a toy store?

When was the last time you drove on grass?

Whose home did you last visit?

When were you last in a different time zone?

When did you last go downtown?

When was the last time someone asked you for help?

When were you last on a train?

When was the last time someone helped you to your feet?

When did you last use a dust pan?

What was the last time you used a suction cup?

Where was the last place you swam that had a lifeguard?

What was the last thing you added to your keychain?

When was the last time you ate in a cafeteria?

When was the last time you drank champagne?

When was the last time you used a spray bottle?

Who was the last friend you added on Facebook?

When was the last time you went to the top of a really tall building?

When was the last time you swallowed a pill?

When was the last time you walked on carpet?

When was the last time you were in an antique shop?

When did you last wear a helmet?

What was the last thing you lost?

When did you last sit on the ground?

When was the last time you operated a jewelry clasp?

When were you last inside an RV?

When did you last use a fork?

What was the last book you looked through at a bookstore but didn't buy?

When was the last time you used a scanner?

When was the last time you were in a shed?

When was the last time your hands touched each other?

When was the last time you walked over a mile?

When was the last time you spoke to your neighbor on the left?

When was the last time someone directed you to turn to a certain page of a book?

When was the last time you heard an outdoor warning siren being tested?

When was the last time you overslept?

When did you last hear the word <u>masterpiece</u>?

When was the last time you played the getting warmer, getting colder game to find something?

What was your game piece for the last board game you played?

When was the last time you tried to make a Slinky go down the stairs?

When was the last time you said out loud who your best friend is?

What happened on this day last month?

When was the last time you put your arm around someone's shoulders?

When did you last see an hourglass?

When did you last look at a map?

When was the last time your height was measured?

When was the last time you left your home and went in a different direction than usual?

When did you last eat at McDonald's?

When was the last time you tried to juggle?

When did you last get sunburnt?

When did you last speak to each of your friends?

When was the last time you opened the hood of a vehicle?

When was the last time you were in an electronics store?

When did you last buy a light bulb?

When was the last time you found out someone's age?

When did you last set the time on a clock?

When was the last time someone cracked your back?

When was the last time you heard that someone had a baby?

When was the last time you were in a car and it turned right?

When was the last time you threw a Frisbee?

When was the last time you tried to read something upside down?

When was the last time you tried to use a hula hoop?

When was the last time you put on a bracelet?

When did you last see a bird's nest?

When was the last time you went down to the basement?

When did you last shoot pool?

When did you last swim in a lake?

How did you last donate your time to charity?

When was the last time you stayed home sick from work or school?

When was the last time you filled a vehicle with gas?

When did you last see a ladybug?

When was the last time you cracked open a nut?

When was the last time you went to the doctor?

What was the last shirt you wore that said something on the front?

When was the last time you looked through a microscope?

When was the last time you drew a picture of a tree?

What was the last quote you heard?

What was the last thing you stirred?

When was the last time you used mouthwash?

When did you last see a waterfall?

When did you last go up on your tiptoes?

When was the last time you went to your county courthouse?

When was the last time you jumped off a diving board?

What was the last building you went into that you had never been in before?

When was the last time you went to the bathroom in an outhouse?

When was the last time you folded a piece of paper?

When was the last time you wore black socks?

When did you last eat Jell-O?

When was the last time you played musical chairs?

When was the last time you wore a blindfold?

When was the last time you used an eraser?

What was the last thing you flipped with a spatula?

When did it last snow?

When was the last time you saw two people try to pay the same bill at a restaurant?

What was the last metal item you bent?

Who was the last person you heard play the guitar?

When was the last time you stepped in dog poop?

When was the last time you listened to a speech?

When did you last play Pac-Man?

Who was the last person you kissed?

When did you last wear a backpack?

When was the last time you spoke to a lawyer?

When was the last time someone was talking on a phone and passed the phone to you?

When did you last ride in a truck?

What was the last thing you threw away in an outdoor trash?

When did you last see sheet music?

What was the last thing you acted out for a game of charades?

When was the last time someone asked to see your driver's license?

When was the last time you couldn't read someone's handwriting?

When did you last shoot a bow and arrow?

When was the last time you used eye drops?

When did the weather last spoil your plans?

When did you last hear a computerized voice?

When did you last take off your shoes?

When did you last wear earplugs?

When did you last hear screeching tires?

When did you last press the button at a crosswalk?

When was the last time you completed a survey?

When did you last eat a pretzel?

Where did you last see your cellphone?

When was the last time you hit your shin on something?

When did you last write a check?

When was the last time you played Minesweeper?

When was the last time you sat outside?

When was last time you put a coin in a spiral coin funnel?

When was the last time you broke down a cardboard box?

What was the last thing you cooked on the stove?

When was the last time you were on an airplane?

Who was the last person you spoke to on the phone who was in a different time zone?

When did you last see a mouse?

When was the last time you opened the cabinet beneath the bathroom sink?

Who was the last person to tell you what they did over the weekend?

When was the last time you gave someone a tip?

What was the last thing you ate off a paper plate?

When was the last time you made physical contact with someone?

When was the last time you ate pie?

When did you last open a sealed envelope?

What was the last thing you bought that required assembly?

When did you last wear sunglasses?

When was the last time you yelled?

What was the last movie you rented from a store?

When was the last time you looked at the ceiling?

Who was the last person to come to your door?

When was the last time you ate chicken?

When did you last ride on a golf cart?

When was the last time you played Simon Says?

What was the last thing you ate that was grown in a garden?

When was the last time you used an ice cream scoop?

When were you last outside on a foggy day?

When was the last time you tasted salt water?

When did you last eat grilled cheese?

What was the last thing you bought from a street vendor?

When was the last time you wore a sweater?

When did you last hear music?

When was the last time you sat on a bench?

When did you last hear the word <u>submarine</u>?

When was the last time you were called by a telemarketer?

Who was the last person you lent money?

When was the last time you went to a car dealership?

When was the last time you used a heating pad?

Where did you last see a fountain?

What was the last thing you did that was spontaneous?

When was the last time you burped?

When did you last sign your name on an electronic pad?

Who was the last person you saw that was really tall?

When was the last time someone called you by the wrong name?

What was the last thing you drank?

When did you last go across a bridge in a vehicle?

What was the last piece of furniture you moved?

When did you last use a gift card?

What was the last CD you listened to?

When was the last time you squeezed a stress ball?

What was the last tattoo you noticed?

When were you last summoned for jury duty?

When was the last time you put a collar on a pet?

When did you last throw a football?

When was the last time you changed a diaper?

When did you last open a desk drawer?

When was the last time you ate a chocolate from a box of chocolates?

When were you last lying down?

When was the last time you set a table?

When did you last go to the grocery store?

What was the last thing you put in your back pocket?

When was the last time you heard the word <u>billion</u>?

When did you last run your fingers through your hair?

When was the last time you kneeled?

When did you last open a safe?

When did you last see a wet floor sign?

What was the last pop-up book you opened?

When was the last time you got a flat tire?

When was the last time you had to get an animal to swallow medicine?

When did you last play darts?

When was the last time you were in a cemetery?

When was the last time you recorded a video?

When did you last see a pig?

When did you last charge your cellphone?

When was the last time you tried to find your way in the dark?

When was the last time you sat on a beanbag?

When was the last time you passed road construction?

When did you last lie on the floor?

When was the last time you jumped on a bed?

What was the last thing you held in your hand?

When was the last time you parked in a parking ramp?

When did you last see a tree stump?

When was the last time you touched your elbow with your hand?

When was the last time you turned on your high-beam headlights?

When was the last time you heard someone do an impression?

When was the last time you found shade to stay cool?

When did you last eat spaghetti?

When was the last time you were in a garage?

When was the last time somebody tried to scare you?

When did you last get a temporary tattoo?

What was the last thing you laminated?

What was the last thing you were shown how to do?

When was the last time you went on a hay rack ride?

When did you last use a Q-tip?

Who was the last person you arm wrestled?

What was the last thing you picked up off the ground?

When was the last time you put a vehicle in neutral?

When did you last buy wrapping paper?

When was the last time you cleared your throat?

What was the last comic book you read?

When was the last time you tracked a cord to its source and/ or destination?

When was the last time you used a laser pointer?

When was the last time you were out of breath?

When was the last time you drank pop?

When was the last time you saw a rubber ducky?

What was the last new hobby you tried?

When did you last cut your fingernails?

When was the last time you got a parking ticket?

When was the last time you spread butter on something?

What happened last Sunday?

Who was the last person to touch your feet?

When was the last time you wore a button-down shirt?

When was the last time you played badminton?

When was the last time you opened a baby gate?

When was the last time you turned on a water faucet?

When did you last hear the word <u>king</u>?

What was the last appetizer you ordered?

When was the last time you got your luggage from baggage claim at an airport?

When was the last time you had a canker sore?

When did you last see a spider?

When was the last time you saw something written on a dirty car?

When was the last time you put on your coat?

When was the last time you touched a tree?

When did you last sit on patio furniture?

When was the last time you heard the word <u>gullible</u>?

What was the last package you received in the mail?

When was the last time you saw a lipstick stain?

When was the last time you were inside a coffee shop?

Where did you last see stained glass?

What was the last candy bar you ate?

When was the last time you used aluminum foil?

When did you last breathe through your mouth?

When did you last see one of your cousins?

When was the last time you had heartburn?

When was the last time you introduced two people to each other?

When was the last time you went snorkeling?

What was the last remote-control toy you operated?

When was the last time your palms were sweaty?

When was the last time you played Marco Polo?

When was the last time you waved your arms to catch someone's attention?

When did you last hear your mother's maiden name spoken aloud?

What was the last app you downloaded?

What happened last Friday?

What was the last test you took?

When did you last use a cutting board?

When was the last time you got lost?

When did you last hear a vehicle beep as it backed up?

What was the last thing you brought to a potluck?

When was the last time you bought a bag of ice?

What was the last thing you got off the top of a refrigerator?

When was the last time you cut something out of a newspaper?

When was the last time you played dodgeball?

When was the last time you fell asleep in a car?

When was the last time you saw an ant?

Where did you last see a marching band perform?

When was the last time you rode a roller coaster?

When was the last time you ate a salad?

When did you last ride a horse?

When was the last time you threw away spoiled food?

When was the last time you wore sandals?

When was the last time you woke up with a sore neck?

When was the last time you threw a snowball at someone?

When was the last time you found a loose hair?

When was the last time you hit the snooze button on an alarm?

When did you last get into a pillow fight?

When was the last time you ate a brownie?

When was the last time you felt a plant to see if it was real?

When was the last time you used tongs?

Who was the last person to bring you a souvenir from their travels?

When was the last time you talked to someone on speakerphone?

When did you last go to the library?

When was the last time you played Ping-Pong?

When was the last time you picked a flower?

When was the last time you took your vehicle to a mechanic?

When was the last time you were on a gravel road?

When was the last time you dimmed a light?

What did you wear last St. Patrick's Day?

When did you last go to the bank?

When was your cholesterol last checked?

When was the last time you used a cotton ball?

What happened last Tuesday?

When was the last time you opened a combination lock?

When did you last eat rice?

When did you last see a balloon get loose outside and fly up into the sky?

When did you last see a globe?

When was the last time you stuck out your tongue at someone?

When did you last say something in a different language?

What was the last book you bought?

When did you last hear the word <u>octopus</u>?

When did you last look in a mirror?

When was the last time you played Hangman?

When was the last time a stranger asked you to take a picture for them?

When did you last use a knife?

When did you last sweat?

When was the last time you had ringing in your ears?

When did you last see a bee?

When was the last time you caught a snowflake on your tongue?

When did you last hear someone play the piano?

When was the last time you rode in a limousine?

What was your last thought before you fell asleep last night?

What was the last carnival game you played?

When was the last time you used duct tape?

When did you last use a throat spray?

When was the last time you used a measuring spoon?

When was the last time you saw a car show?

When did you last open one of the drawers in the refrigerator?

When was the last time you accidentally called someone by the wrong name?

When did you last hang your coat on a hook?

When was the last time you were placed in alphabetical order by name?

When did you last play Uno?

When was the last time you entered a password?

When did you last use a bottle opener?

When did you last eat a Girl Scout cookie?

When did you last hear a first name that you had never heard before?

When did you last see an aquarium?

When were you last given a receipt?

When did you last eat cottage cheese?

What was the last movie poster you saw?

When was the last time you interlocked your fingers?

When was the last time you ate Skittles?

When was the last time your teeth chattered?

What was the last thing you had dry cleaned?

When was the last time you took bottles or cans to a redemption center?

When was the last time you wiped your feet?

When was the last time you bluffed?

When did you last open your wallet?

When did you last touch the floor with your hand?

When was the last time you were in a vehicle moving in reverse?

When did you last look out a window?

When was the last time you used a touch-screen device?

When did you last open the bottom drawer of your dresser?

When did you last use a pen?

When was the last time you sat on a lawn chair?

When was the last time you untangled a knot?

When was the last time you played tennis?

When did you last type a question mark?

When did you last hear your smoke detector go off?

When was the last time you ate grapes?

When was the last time you wound a music box?

Who was the last person you borrowed money from?

What was the last thing you bought off a wedding registry?

What was the last phone number you looked up?

When was the last time you used an ATM?

When was the last time you saw a dunk tank?

When was the last time you got stitches?

What was the last new food you tried?

What was the last magazine you bought?

When was the last time a repairperson came to your home?

When did you last see a deer?

When was the last time you colored an Easter egg?

When was the last time you accidentally left your to-go container at a restaurant?

When was the last time you bought a raffle ticket?

When was the last time you opened a box that was taped shut?

What was the subject line of your last email?

When was the last time _____?

ABOUT THE AUTHOR

Matthew Welp was born and raised in Norwalk, Iowa. He attended Creighton University in Omaha, Nebraska, where he earned a Doctor of Pharmacy degree. After graduation, Matthew returned to Iowa, where he met his amazing wife, Whitney. Matthew wrote "When Was the Last Time?" when he was 30 years old. The writing of it had a lot to do with his grandpa, a wonderful man who passed away in 2007 after a tough battle with dementia. Through the ups and downs, Matthew is grounded by his family. He is uplifted by his friends. He is inspired by Whitney.

Printed in the United States
By Bookmasters